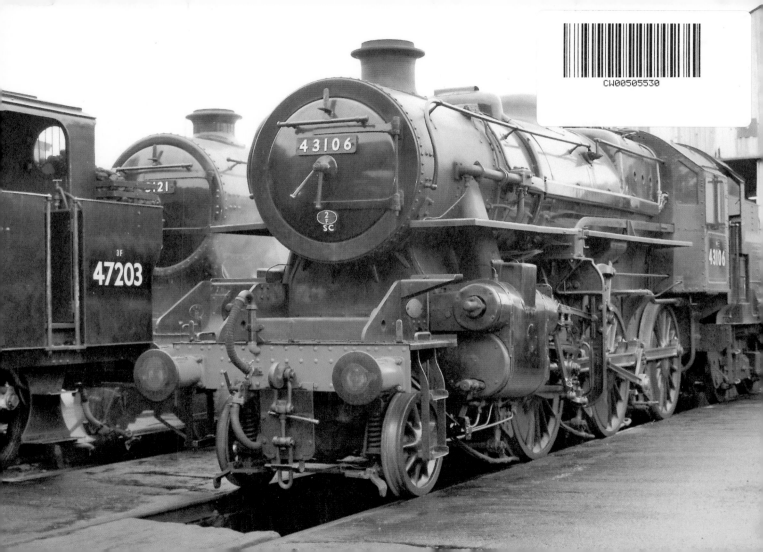

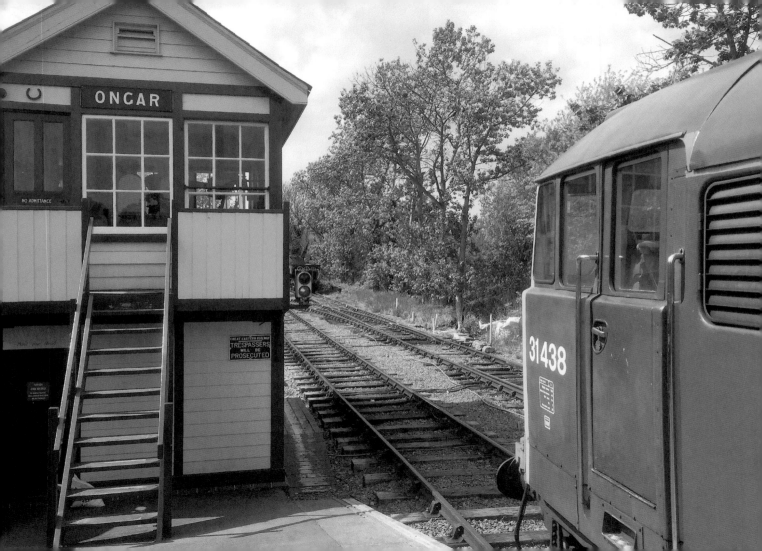

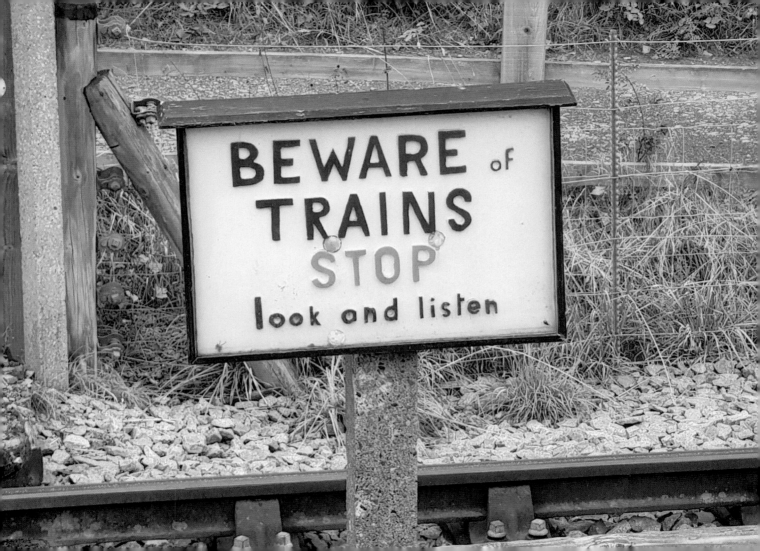

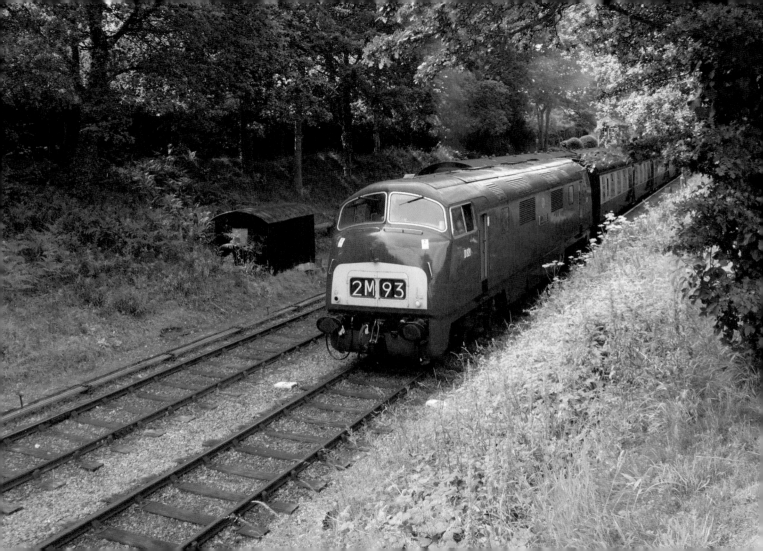

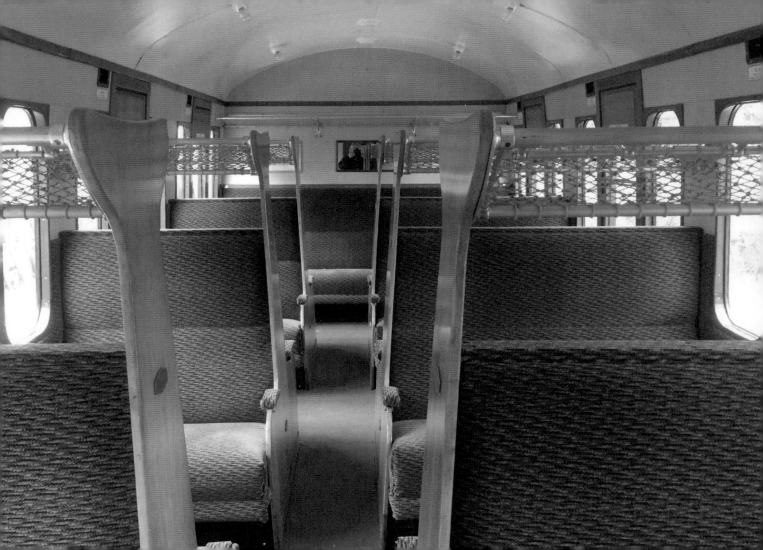

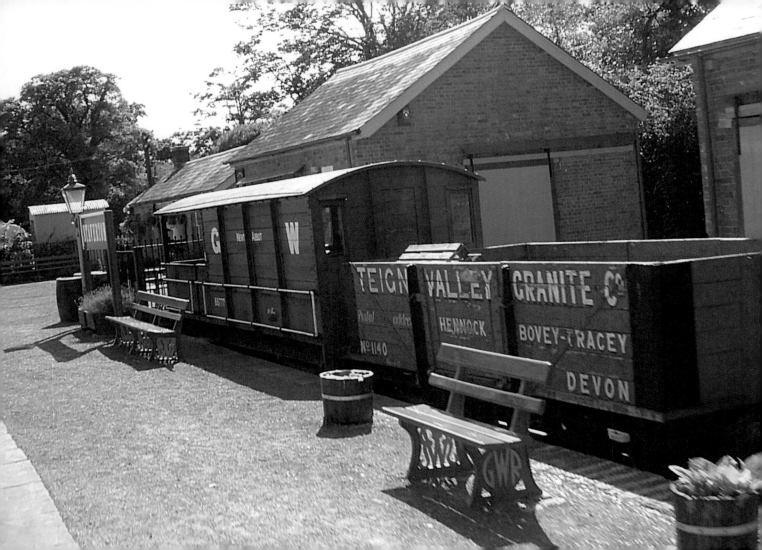

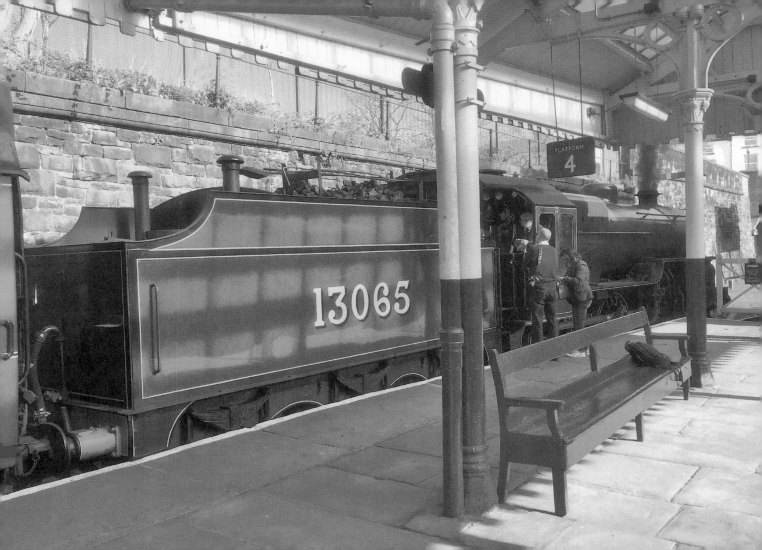

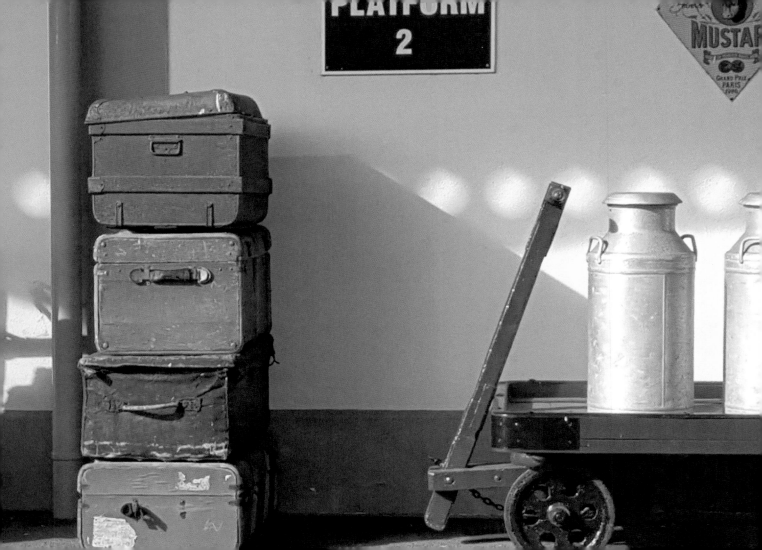

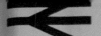

Passenger Timetable
6 May 1974 to 4 May 1975

Great Britain
Inter-City, local and suburban services
Irish, Channel Islands, Coastal services

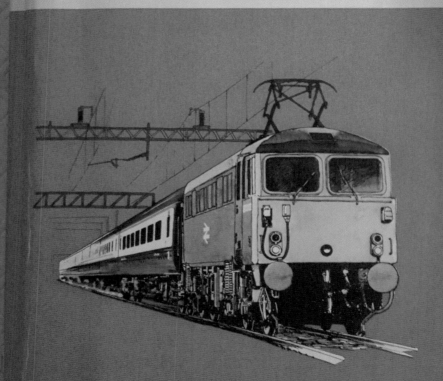

50p

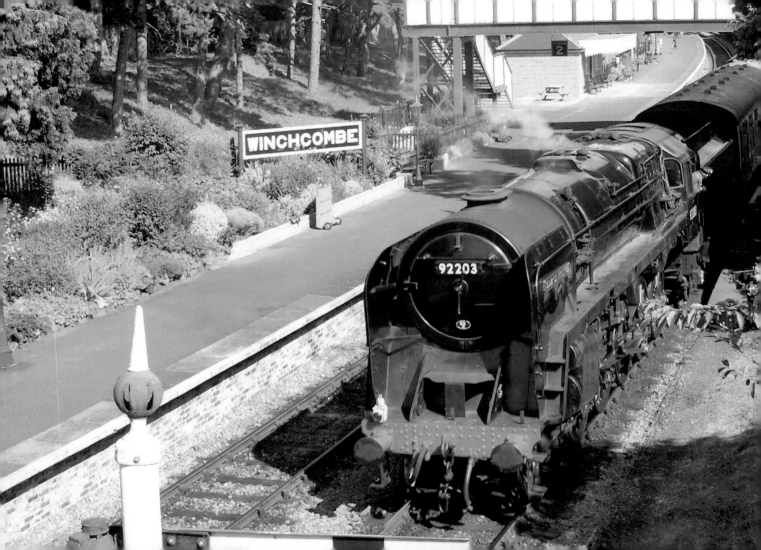

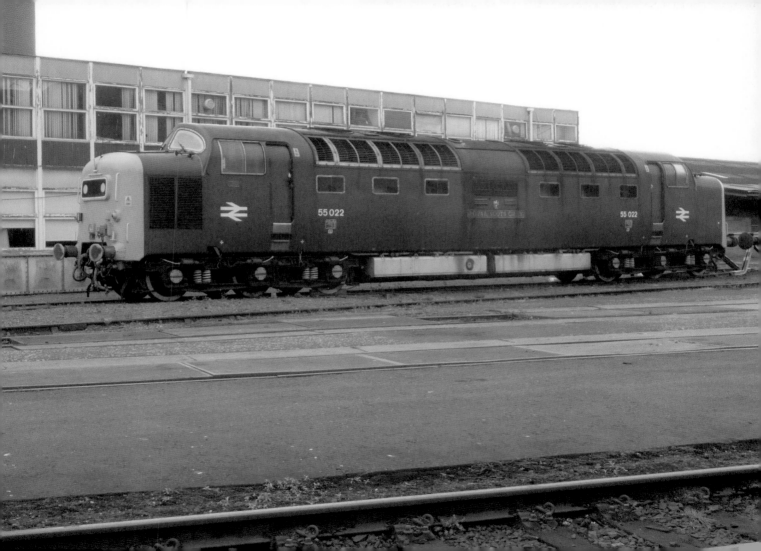

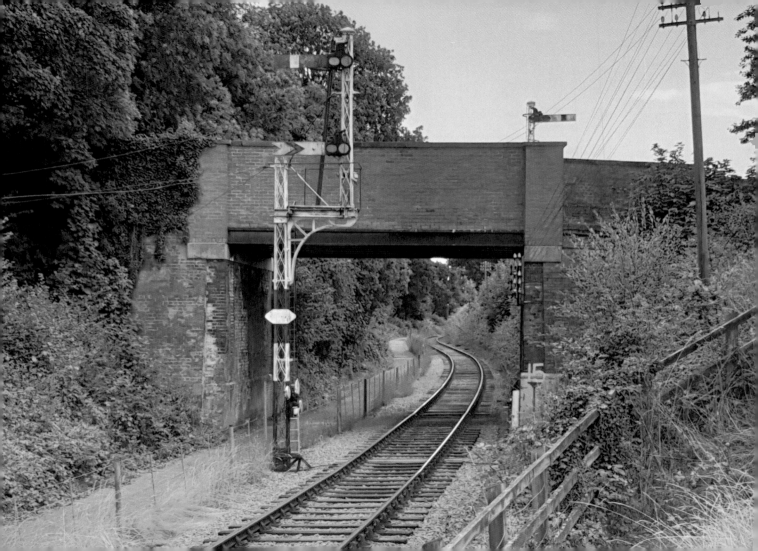

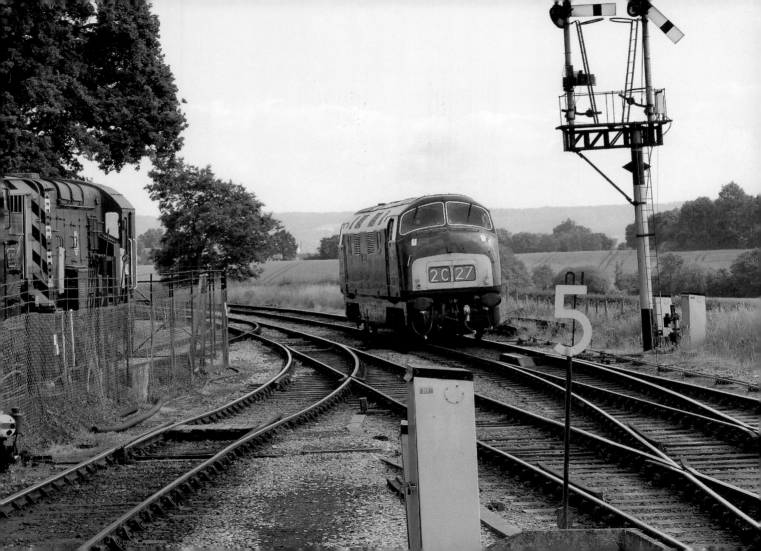

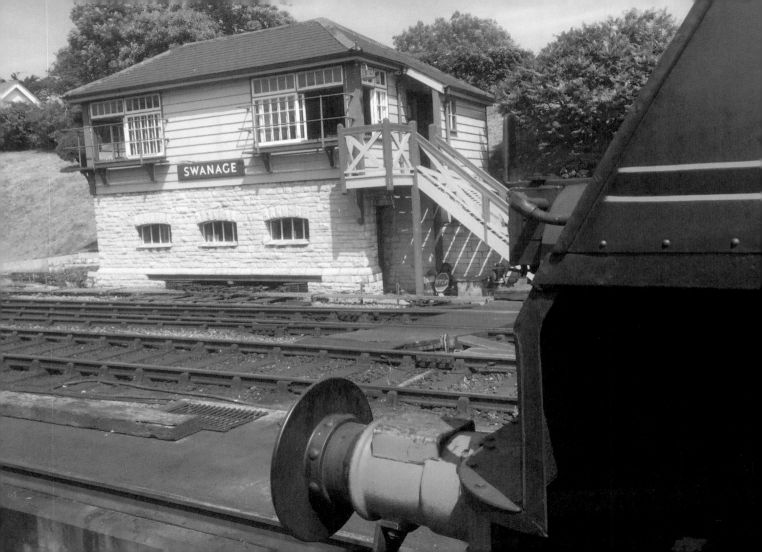

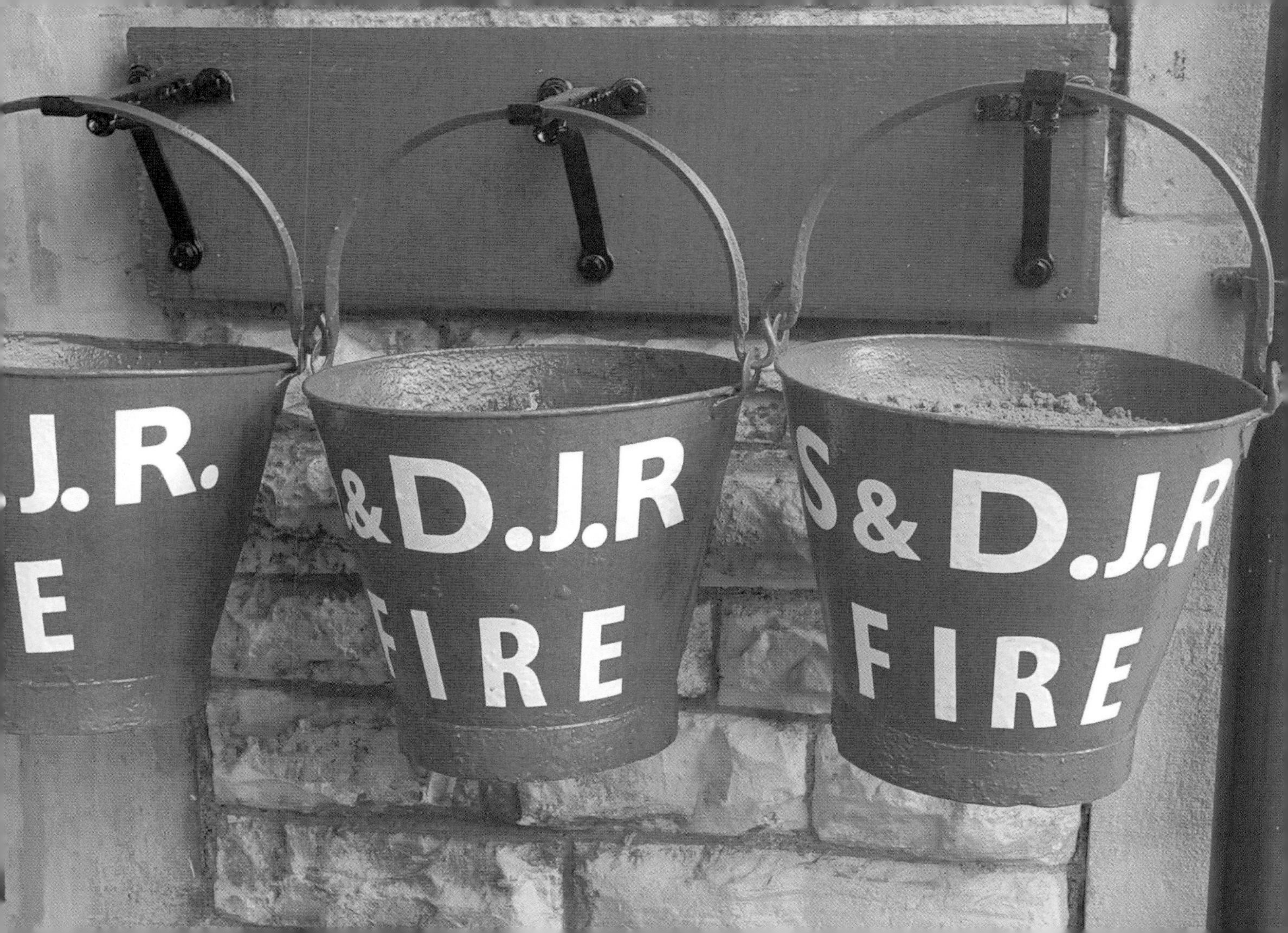

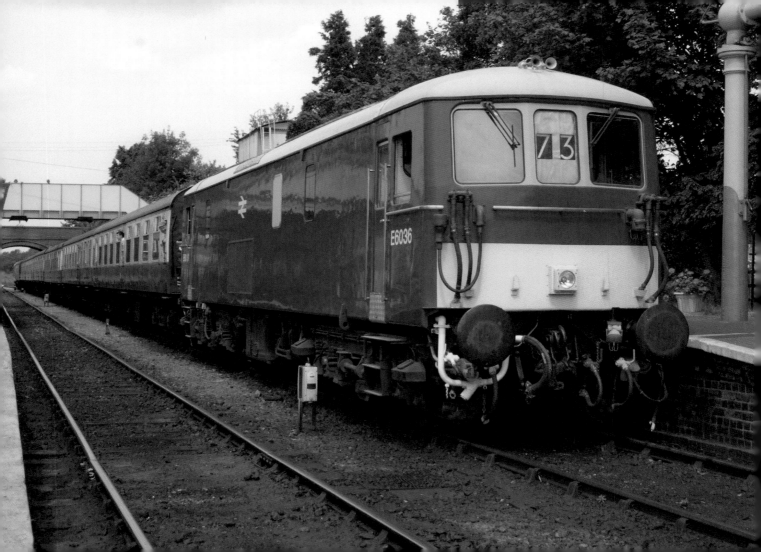

3142	2nd - CHEAP DAY	CHEAP - 2nd DAY	3142
	Cambridge to STEVENAGE	Stevenage to CAMBRIDGE	
	(E) For conditions see over	For conditions see over (E)	

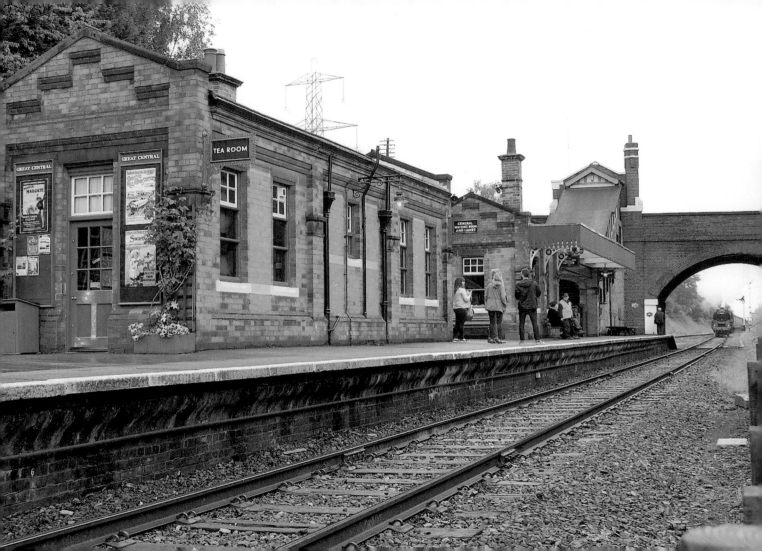

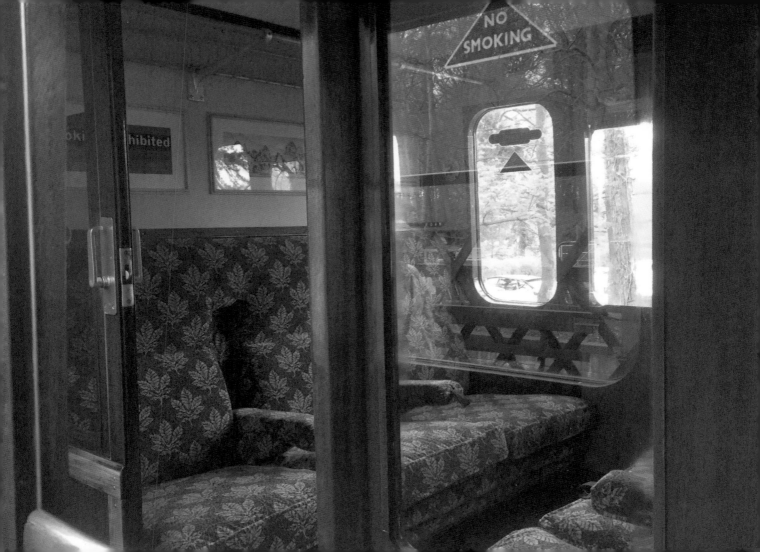

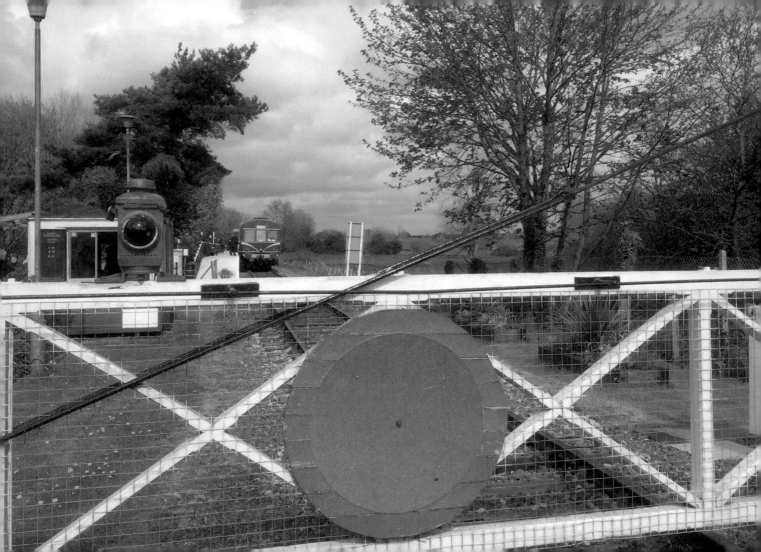

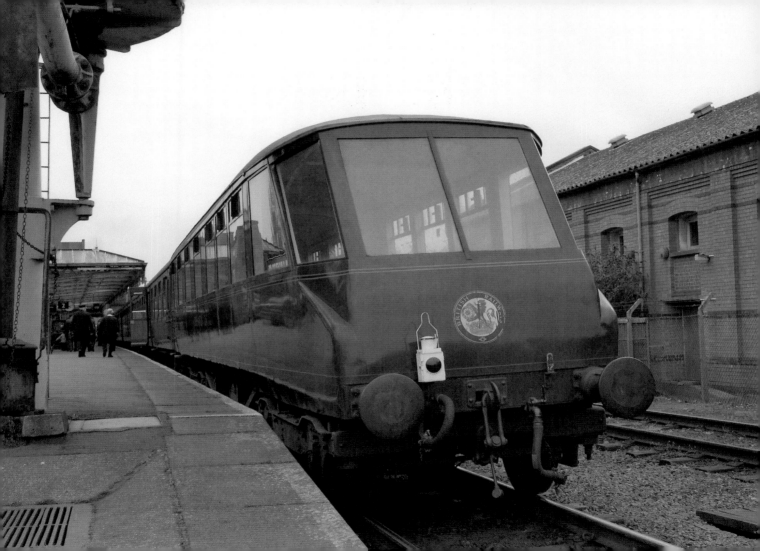

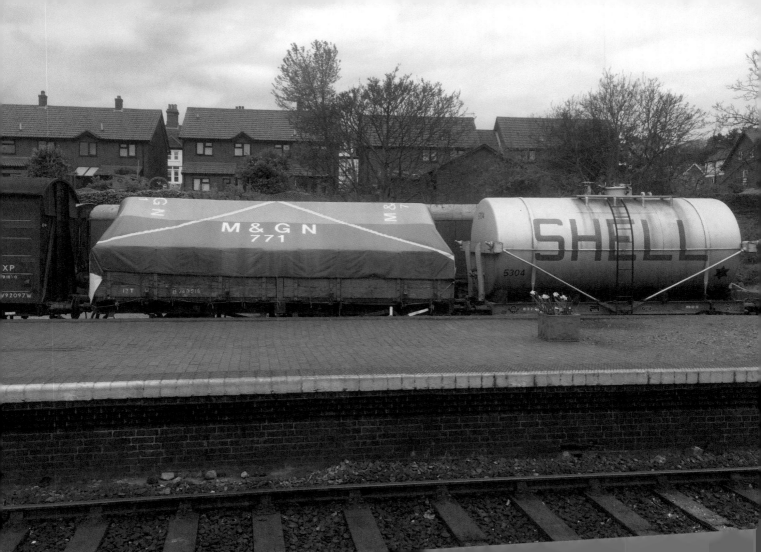

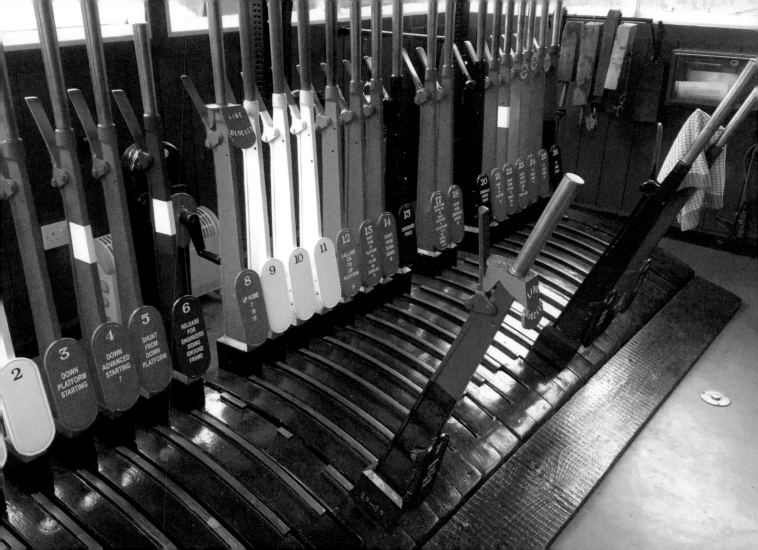

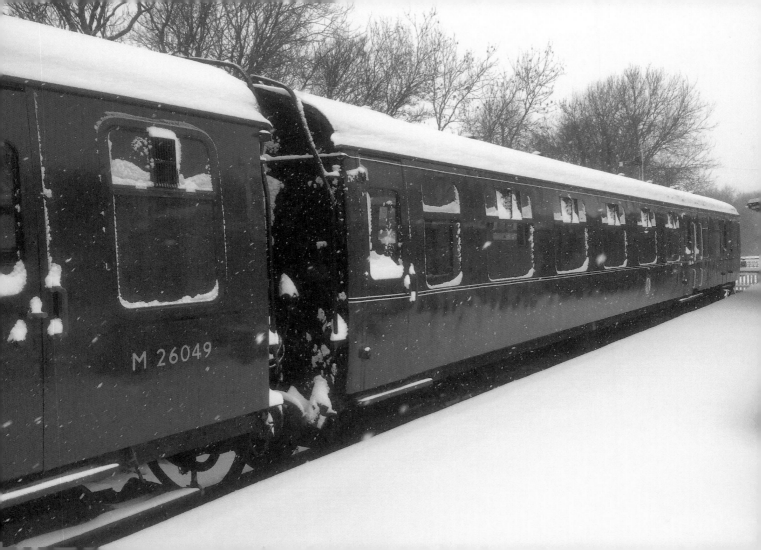

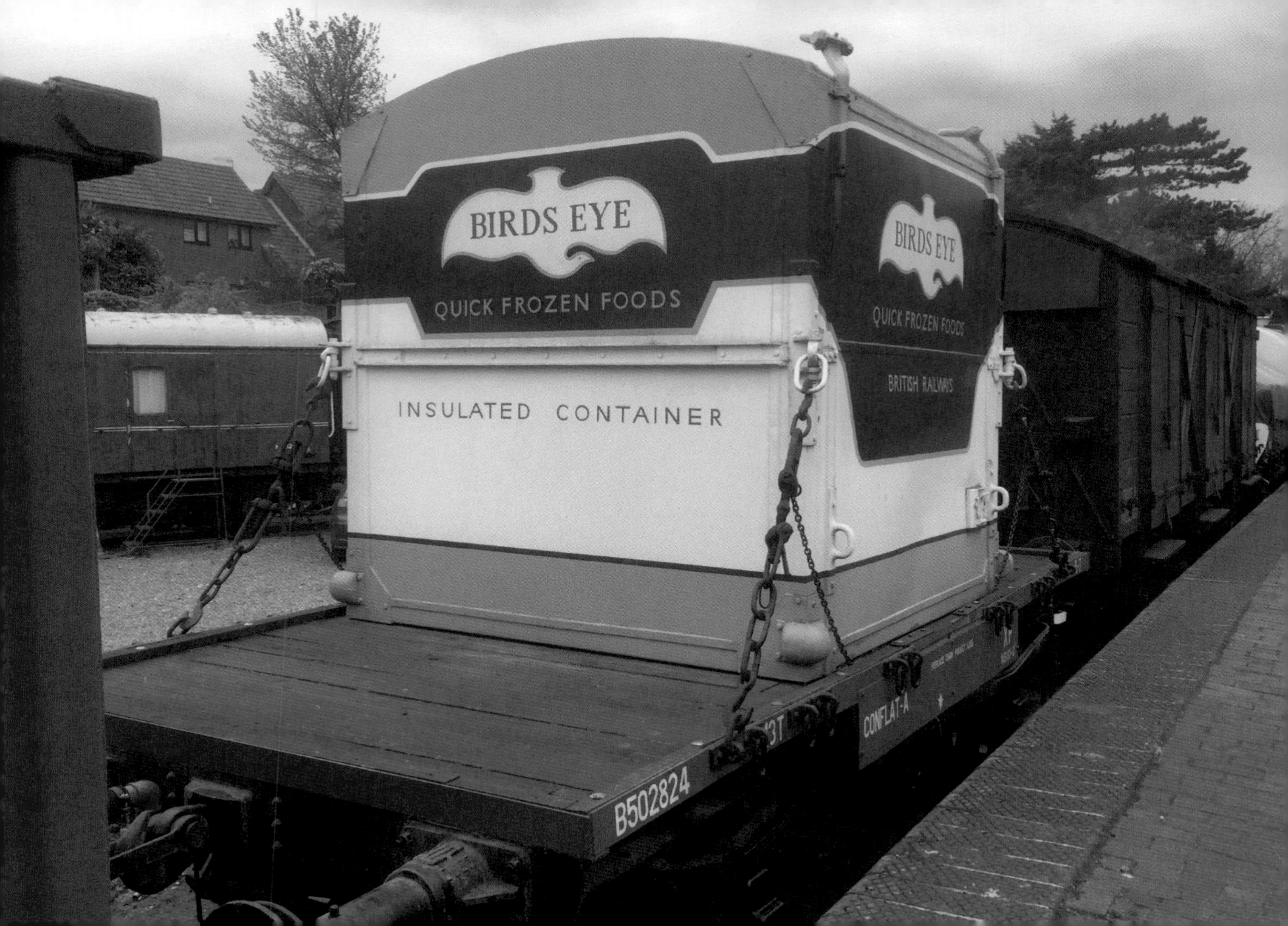
BIRDS EYE
QUICK FROZEN FOODS
INSULATED CONTAINER
BIRDS EYE
QUICK FROZEN FOODS
BRITISH RAILWAYS
CONFLAT-A
B502824

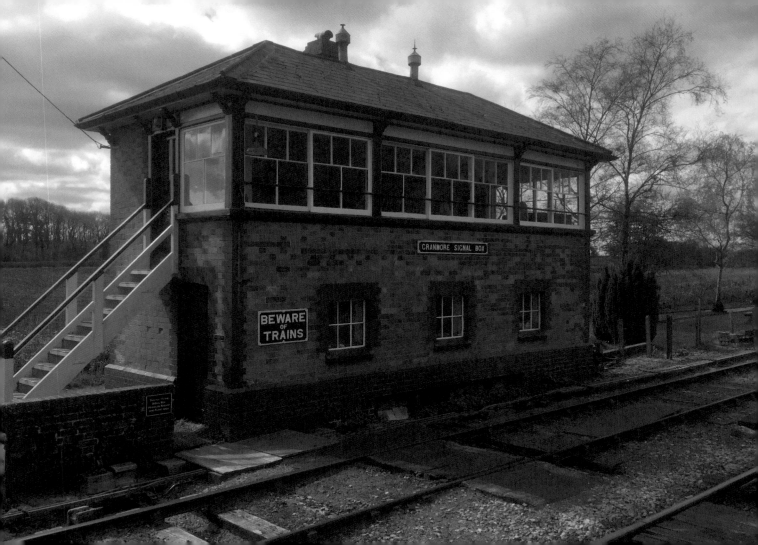

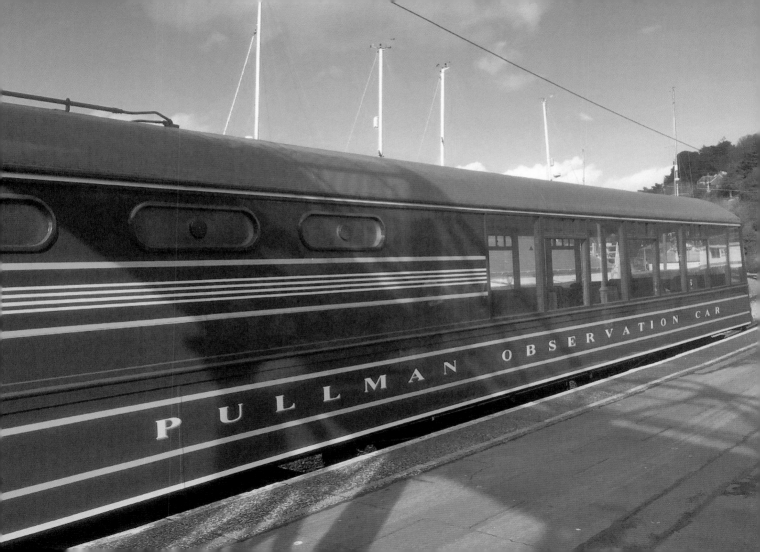

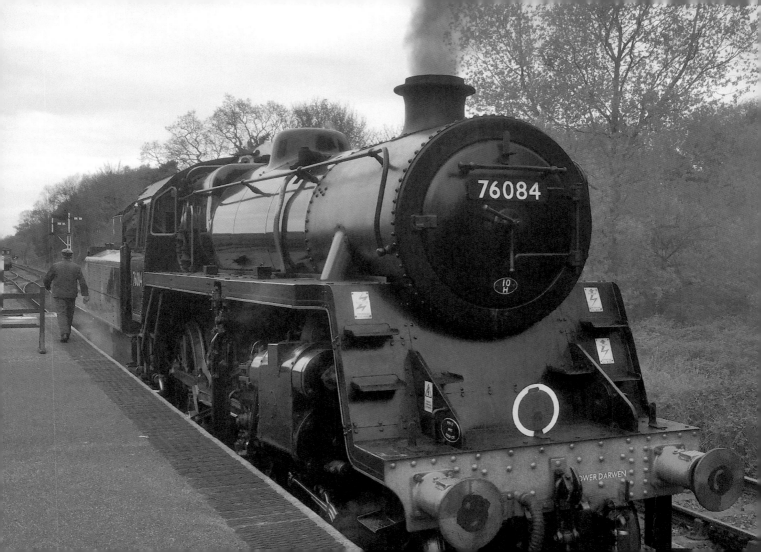

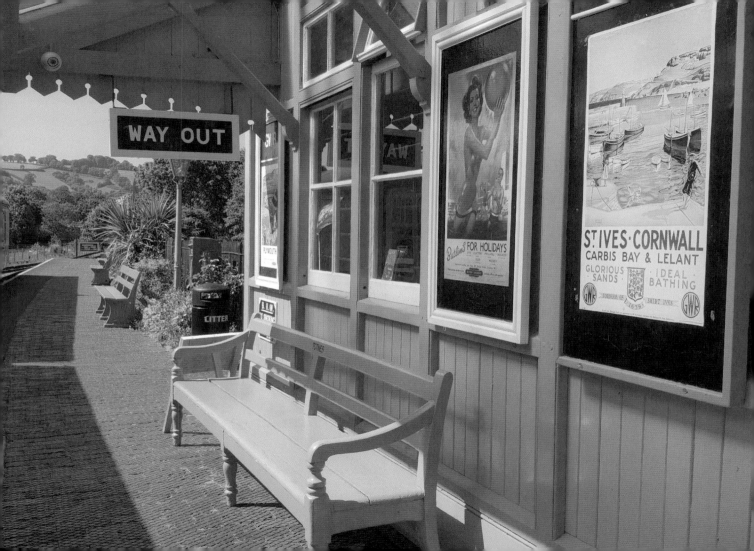

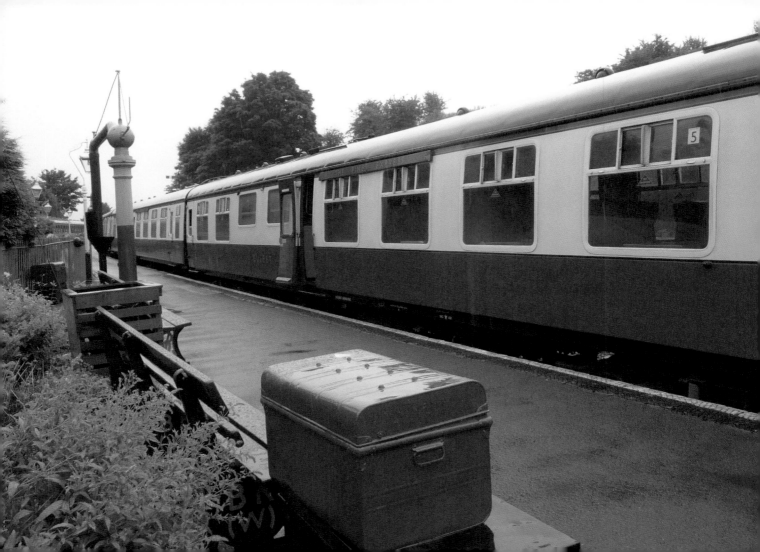

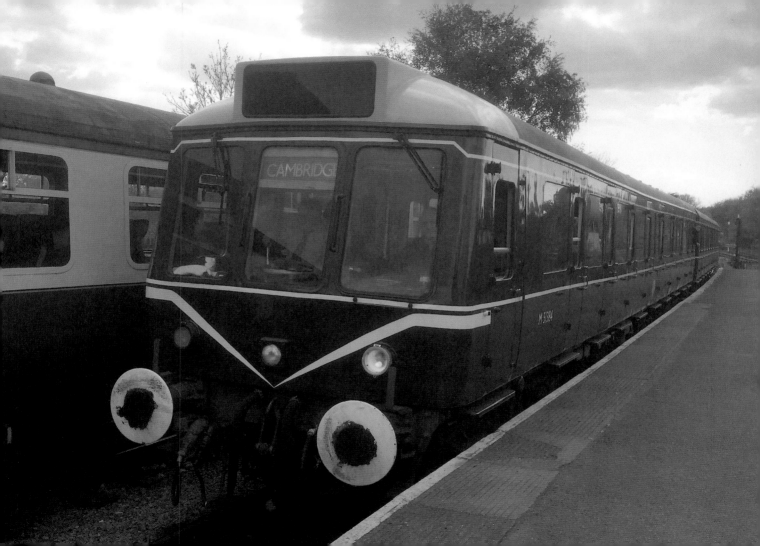

The Broads

Wide lagoons much loved by yachtsmen, linked by peaceful rivers and canals. In all, more than 200 miles of water. At busy Oulton Broad, the southern gateway, visitors will find much natural beauty and every facility that could reasonably be expected. Including some of the finest coarse angling you'll find anywhere, with tackle available for hire. Somewhere quieter? Try the charm of Wroxham, Horning or Potter Heigham and relax a little in the comforting atmosphere of one of the many riverside inns.

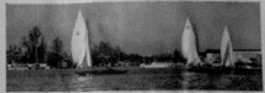
The Broads

Ely

Dominated by its magnificent Norman cathedral, this town is in the heart of a district known as the 'Isle of Ely'. Centuries ago, Ely really was an island amongst the undrained fens, and it was from here that Hereward the Wake defied William the Conqueror long after the Normans had overruled the rest of the country. Today Ely is an island in name only and offers a serene welcome to the visitor. But a few hundred acres of fens have been preserved as a nature reserve around Wicken.

In addition to Great Yarmouth, seaside resorts waiting to welcome you include Cromer and Felixstowe.

You can get your Anglian Ranger from any Inter-City station in the area or from your travel agent. They're available from 17th May to 25th September 1971 and you can use them each day (but only from 08.45 onwards on Monday to Friday). Your ticket gives you 7 days unlimited travel anywhere in East Anglia for only £2.

Take a holiday soon. By Anglian Ranger

Your Travel Agent

Published by British Rail Eastern

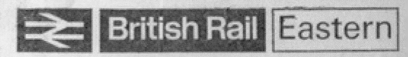

British Rail Eastern

2nd CLASS   **Rate £1.00**

ANGLIAN RANGER

Valid from   **2 9 JUL 1972**

Until   **04 AUG 1972**

VALID AS ADVERTISED

Available at stations shown on back

NOT Valid before 0845 on Mondays

to Fridays

Signature of holder   *Barrie Pepperworth*

FOR CONDITIONS ENQUIRE AT TICKET OFFICE

This Ticket is NOT
TRANSFERABLE
and must be given
up on expiry

Nᵒ _ 1910

BR. 3501/47

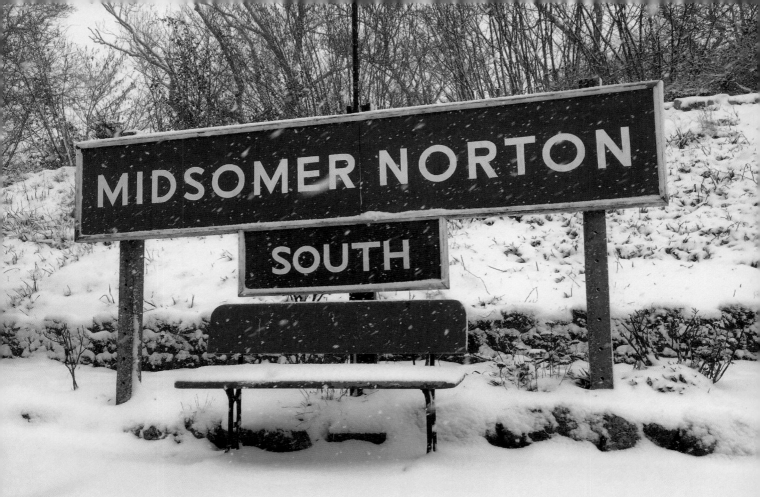

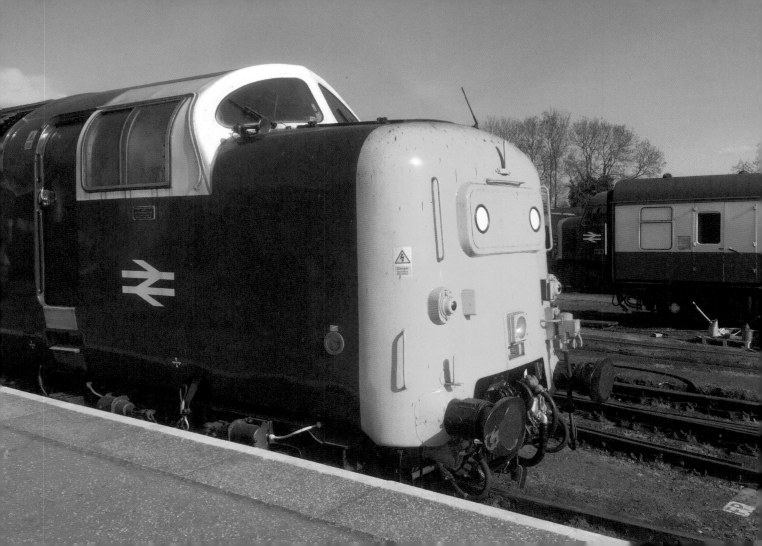

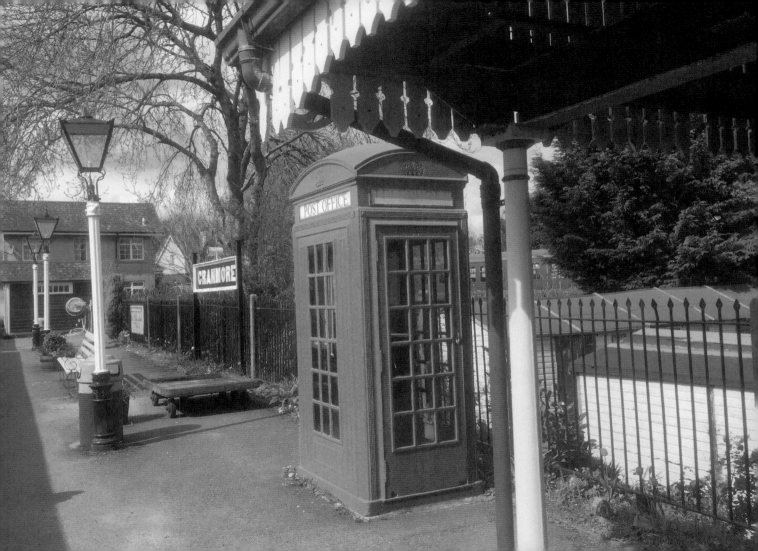

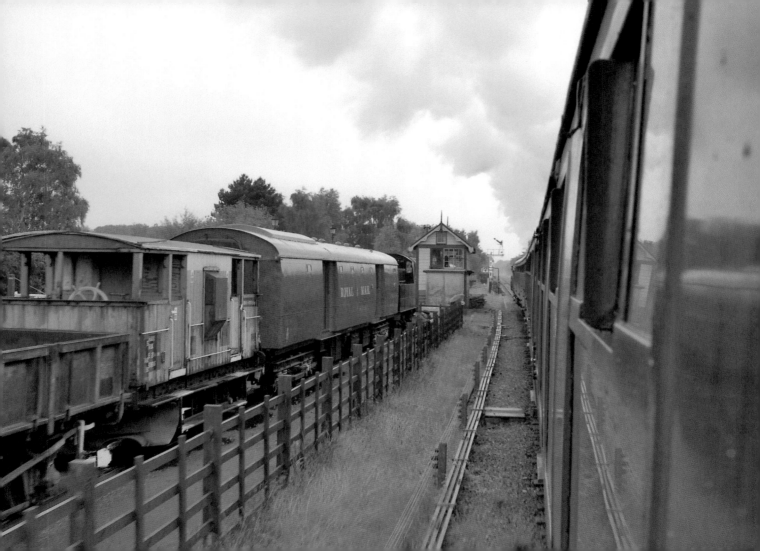

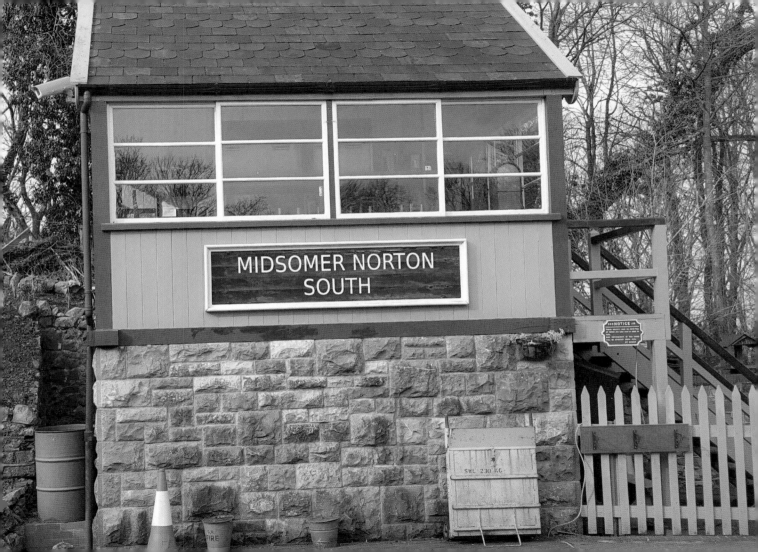

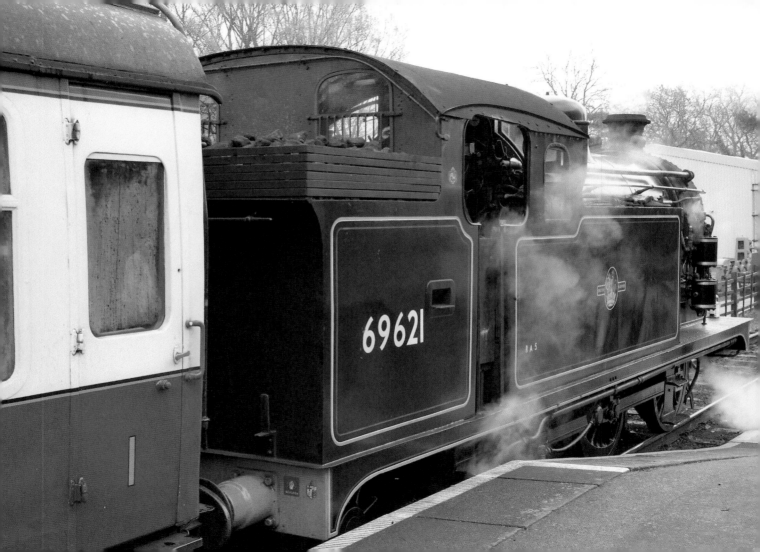

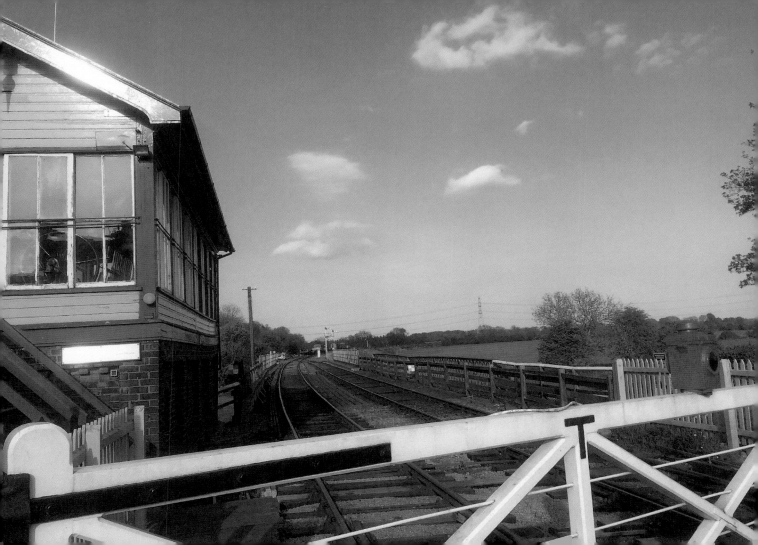

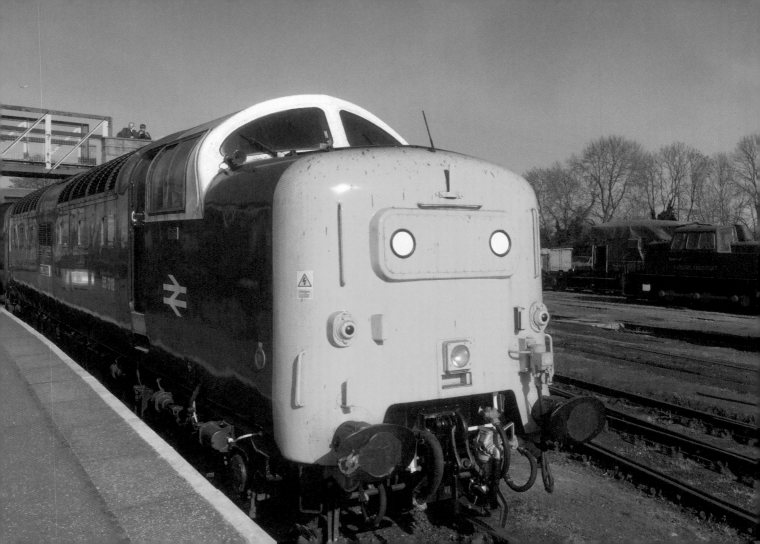

Printed in Great Britain
by Amazon